Hi Cancer,
I'm listening

Dr CLARE MUNDAY

1	Preface by author	p. 5
1.1	Preface by Dr Hamid Montakab	p. 10
1.2	Acknowledgments	p. 17
2	Introduction	p. 19
3	Cancer, who are you ?	p. 26
3.1	Cancer, what's your name ?	p. 29
3.2	What does science say of You ?	p. 31
4	Cancer, how dare you knock on my door ?	p. 34
4.1	Are You a punishment ?	p. 37
4.2	Hey Cancer, could I've avoided You ?	p. 39
4.3	The Truth	p. 41
4.4	Have You given me warning signs ? What do You have to say to me ?	p. 43

5   Cancer, what am I   p. 45
        going to do with You ?

5.1   What are the heavy   p. 47
        treatments to knock
        You out ?

5.2   What are the soft   p. 52
        options for getting rid of
        You ?

5.3   What are Your thoughts   p. 63
        on food ?

5.4   Is my life style   p. 67
        important ?

5.5   Listening to yourself, to p. 69
        Me and to your body

5.6   What about emotions ?   p. 72

5.7   Is there a place for   p. 74
        guides, and guardian
        angels ?

6   And when You come   p. 78
        back ?

7   When I win the game,   p. 80
        what do You do ?

7.1   What does winning really mean ?   p. 81

8   Can I live with You ?   p. 82

9   Death   p. 85

9.1   Suffering, fatigue, pain and palliative care   p. 88

10   Conclusion   p. 94

11   Suggested readings   p. 96

1 Preface by author

This book is dedicated to all the beings who have helped me awaken, including and especially, Cancer itself. Throughout my career as a medical oncologist, I've been lucky to meet the "right sort of people". They have shown me the way, the good sides and the pitfalls. They have challenged me and enhanced my thought processes, guided me and shown me different ways of thinking. To see the many possibilities and the unusual paths, especially those that are less explored. Cancer is such a revealer of truths that this is what ultimately inspired me to write this unusual book.

I remember very clearly a young patient with a very large tumour of the underside of the tongue, whose chances of healing, both medical and scientific, were very poor, and who wanted to be OK with his cancer ... So he found a therapist who helped him negotiate, between the cancer and himself, to reach a consensus ... He got cured, to my astonishment, despite medical treatment that would be today considered as massively sub-optimal. From then on and for several years, I saw this man walking to and fro in front of my practice in search of the next steps; he had faced his illness but, after all, he had clearly not found meaning in his life even though he had come very close to death. He even wondered why it had happened to him. To him and his therapist, thank you, they opened another path for me, that of the negotiation with the parts of oneself, where cancer is a part, using techniques such as NLP(neuro linguistic programming). Without them, I would never have known that this way ahead existed.

On the other hand, I have also learnt that healing from a serious, potentially life-threatening illness, does not necessarily make you happy nor give meaning to one's life. A young patient, after his physical healing, "berated me» (rather nicely, I must say), and then sank into a drastic alcohol abuse that killed him a few years later. He longed for this death, and at each follow-up consultation spoke about it. I reminded him that it was together that we had chosen the medical treatment regimens, yet he attributed his healing to the good care of medicine and me in this context. He could not imagine that there was a connection between his life, his cure from cancer and his overall condition .... No treatment or care could help him to overcome his anger and sadness at having become a "long survivor" of cancer. The price to pay is sometimes harsh and difficult, not only emotionally, but because the long-term side effects often worsen progressively with time and they became crippling for this man who lost completely faith in himself and in life.

The side effects of our "classical" oncological treatments are often largely underestimated by the medical and scientific community. They are not always predictable despite our immense knowledge. Statistics remain statistics and the human being cannot be described by statistics. Evaluating a person's personal risk of complications or long-term side effects is very difficult in medicine, and is even more difficult for the physician and the human beings that we are.

I therefore concluded that living was not necessarily the only option, and that death as a possible outcome should be broadly discussed upstream, at the time of diagnosis along with the potential side effects of treatment modalities. And this, even if the prognosis and the therapeutic chances of survival were excellent. However, even discussed widely, the positioning difficulties of the sick human are not simple. The pressure of survival at all costs, is so strong in our society.

The human being is only a kind of materialistic machine that we repair. The more global sense of the experiences we live is often completely overshadowed by this pressure to heal and maintain life at all costs.

Ours is a complex post-industrial society, which favors healing willy-nilly, without taking into account the global context and the people behind. The notion of meaning in our lives has disappeared. Death being part of our lives even more so. A holistic vision is therefore needed to avoid, as much as possible, the pitfalls such as those mentioned above. It is this broad approach that patients and cancer have taught me, and sometimes the need to rely on other forces, the so-called spiritual forces, all but forgotten in our materialistic world. The notion of a soul path that is not necessarily with the body must also be taken into account despite the difficulties of this approach.

This book looks at Cancer as a being in its own right that often interferes with our lives, while never leaving us indifferent. From there, the idea of listening to It and writing a book taken from the point of view of Cancer itself. Cancer is still, today, such a master for me and a for a group

of conscious and "enlightened" humans, that it is no longer possible, well into the 21 first century, to consider oncological disease as due to " bad luck "or as a "punishment" for over indulging in drink, smoking, sunbathing, or rich food, or for having been in contact with   toxic products or the like.
The complexity of this "Cancer being intertwined with its human being" is far beyond our simplistic visions: I change a spare part, do the repair and eureka, I'm on the way off again.

1.1 Preface by Dr Hamid Montakab

Traditional Chinese Medicine (TCM) considers the human as a three-dimensional being: physical, energetic (vibrational) and psycho-spiritual.

Our allopathic medicine has primarily explored the physical dimensions (anatomic and biochemical), which has resulted in an impressive progress in the fields of pharmacology, surgery with a great impact on diagnosis and therapy. Quite naturally, this therapeutic approach reflects our Western thinking and belief systems, which are the results of Cartesian and Newtonian reasoning (cause and effect).

The Western approach differs greatly from the Eastern, in particular the TCM vision, which considers the human in its integral three-dimensional state. According to the TCM concepts, any physical pathology has required a previous energetic disturbance, itself the result of an emotion, a thought process or a "belief". It is very interesting to note that the fields of quantum physics and epigenetics have confirmed many of the ancient Chinese medical concepts in the recent years.

MTC considers that before a disease manifests physically, there will be specific energetic disturbances and pain.

Our body is like a new-born child. To express itself, the infant has only one language, it cries. No matter if the child is hungry, thirsty, in pain, needing its diapers changed or simply asking for attention, it can only cry to attract our attention.

In the same way, our body has only one language and that is "pain".

When we are in pain, our natural reflex is to stop the pain by any means. If the pain resists the usual painkillers, we consult specialists who will explain the origin of our suffering as the result of a physical or a biochemical disturbance. An appropriate treatment is prescribed in the form of an antalgic, anti-inflammatory or some anti…

At times when the allopathic or mechanical medicine has not found a causative factor, a "psycho-somatic" origin is proposed and the search is oriented towards the sub-conscious.

When the inner being continues to suffer and it's pleading for help have not been heard or understood, the body manifests the "disease". When there is an ulcer, a tumor, a hernia or a thrombosis, one cannot ignore this call for help anymore. But allopathic medicine has still more solutions to propose: find and eliminate the culprit at any cost; surgery, radiation or chemical intervention.

The word disease (dis-ease), suggests a "loss of ease". What is it trying to communicate ? Do we wonder how this "ease" was disturbed and lost ?

When our child cries, we try to understand what is the matter and respond to its demands. We do not shut it up. And yet we do precisely this to our poor bodies, we clam it up, ignoring it's calls, and then we are surprised and shocked when we are handed the final diagnosis: it is

CANCER !

I find admirable that Dr. Clare Munday has allowed this infant to express itself. Having had the courage, as an oncologist, to take up the defence of this innocent child who is only pleading to be understood and loved.

Our cancer is not our enemy just the infant within crying for our attention.

In "Hi Cancer, I'm listening", Dr. Munday puts the emphasis precisely on this point: what exactly is my dis-ease telling me ? Thank you, my friend, my dis-ease, for bringing to my attention what has gone astray, what changes I need to make in my life; and most of all, forgive me for having taken so long to hear your call !

As Clare explains, we are not all ready or even equipped to hear the desperate calls of our soul, or to bring about the changes that are required. Fortunately, the allopathic medicine with its drastic measures is there to at least deal with the physical manifestations.

The erroneous belief that "I" am the poor victim of this terrible affliction, that my disease is the result of my wrong life style, environment, or even some divine punishment for my sins, keeps us in a state of dependency. As such we need to be saved either by our medical institution or by divine intervention.

But what if it is "I" am the creator of my disease ? Could I also be the healer ? Yes, this is a very heavy responsibility and we do not all have the strength or the necessary means to shoulder this burden.

At times a good hit on the head can wake us up from our slumber, or else knock us out for good !

Personally, I have had the great fortune to have known both sides, doctor and patient. As a cancer patient, I had to apply my own theories and to change my thinking and belief systems.

And most of all I had to ask and accept help to find my way.

From this rich experience, I would like to share the following points:

No matter what therapy has been chosen, allopathic, alternative, spiritual…, what is most important is to believe in it 100%. Our subconscious does not tolerate doubts.

For example, one belief could be "chemotherapy is a poison…", an alternative belief could be "chemotherapy is a divine nectar…". It is imperative to align our thoughts with the chosen therapy. The mind can be tricky, that is where one has to detect the doubts: "..Yes, but…". When in doubt, ask for outside help; a good therapist may help clarify the thought process.

Even a religious or spiritual belief may be questioned; there is a great difference between "...I believe in you Lord if you save me..." or "...may your will be done..." !

The most difficult challenge is to accept and welcome our disease. My cancer is "me"; rejecting and detesting, it is like hating myself; no different from a suicidal act.

To listen for, to hear the distressing calls of my inner soul is difficult. To take the necessary steps to remedy this suffering is even more difficult.

In my humble opinion, we cannot heal from a serious, life threatening disease by simply picking up our lives as before. One must constantly remember that at some point in our lives, our subconscious had come to a dead-end, and that life, at that moment, had no more sense. This allowed our system to accept the multiplication of anarchic cells. Therefore to continue to live, we will have to learn to say "Yes" to life in the totality of our being.

Finally, the concept of "healing" has to be addressed. From an allopathic point of view, healing is defined by the absence of cancerous cells during the following five years after treatment has ended. But from a spiritual perspective, our disease is but the external manifestation of an inner disease. It is the rift between our conscious mind and our inner soul. True healing is only achieved when we can re-unite the conscious with sub-conscious.

Even if this happens at the very last moment, true healing has been achieved!

The bottom line is: regaining our health is so simple, all it takes is to hear the message of this infant that is crying within….

Thank-you Clare, for your insight and courage.

1.2 Acknowledgments

I thank all those who have worked with me to make this book happen and become public.
As with every creation, it has been an adventure with a long gestational period. It can now take off on its own, meet with love, disenchantment or criticism (be it positive or negative), since it will henceforth have its own life and its own path.

A special thank you to Gilles, my husband, for the layout and editing. Thanks to Bérénice and Nathalie, the fairies who accompany me on this journey as a healer and as a doctor. A big thank for their ideas, proposals, comments and the lively discussions we've often had.
A big thanks you to Diana Miserez for formatting the English version, a great challenge too. This will make for a wider circulation in the English-speaking world. Many thanks to a very dear friend, Cunégonde de Lapoulardière for her help in all ways.

Thank you to you Dr Hamid Montakab for the preface of both the French and the English version. He has walked with this complex being, listened to it and to his heart and moved on in an extraordinary way. I'm greatly moved by what he has said about this book.

Stéphane Marclay has excelled in getting what I wanted in terms of the illustrations and drawings. His cancer cell makes me laugh out loud. I love the cancer cell doctor behind his desk which is usually my place. Just fabulous, I love them; Thanks Stéphane. And if you have a graphic project, he may be happy to develop it with you, just find him on Facebook.

Happy reading, and do write to me if you feel so inclined !

2 Introduction

When I toyed with the idea of writing a new book after a very reasonable and conventional first book on medical approaches in oncology, I wondered what the reader would like to be able to find in another book on such a subject as cancer. It was as I talked to people along the way that the idea of this funny and reflective book came to me !

It was to be challenging and to offer the reader a different and above all wider approach than the classic "my path to healing" or "the ABC of how to conquer cancer" books of which there exists a plethora on the shelves of bookshops.

The goal of this little manual is to approach cancer differently. The subject is, in many minds, intrinsically filled with a lot of anger. For Cancer is terribly frightening to many people, a killer, at least in the collective thought. So I decided to provide a different outlook, more playful, introducing a novel approach.

For almost 30 years, Cancer has shared my path. It's a companion, sometimes a lousy buddy sometimes rebellious but always at the rendez-vous, since I am a medical doctor specialized in oncology. I have therefore rubbed shoulders with It, for better or for worse ! A funny marriage but a marriage anyway.

Cancer is an entity, (and I use this term on purpose and not the term disease) - so variable and so difficult to understand that It remains very mysterious, multi-faceted with unexpected behavior that seems to follow no precise rules. More than once, It will surprise you with Its whimsical know-how. It can be calm or facetious, dangerous or banal but It rarely leaves one indifferent. It is a more and more common "evil" in the Western world as It is currently the first cause of illness and death though a little over 20 years ago this was not the case.

Do you think that It could be, not an enemy to be defeated but another part of oneself, rather strange and bizarre, which speaks a totally different language ? Does It have a point of view and have you given It some of your precious time to listen to this point of view ? After being burned, cut, poisoned, tortured and you with It, does It still have something to reveal about you, about your life, about your life path or even about the meaning of your life ? Is not your body an integral part of yourself ? Is It only in the body ?

And, what if the cancer was there for a reason ? A good or even a bad reason ! And if It was your friend and not a foe ? ... and if by different approaches you could not only tame It but try to understand what It has to say to you ! Not from a scientific point of view but those of other outlooks. Those that come from listening, a listening to you in the depth of your being .... including your pitfalls and impossibilities.

This little book represents a vision which is "avant-garde", and far from the Manichean thoughts of our bio technological society where everything is resolved without listening and without taking into account the core of your being.

What explains that in 2018 the number of cancers is growing, despite all our incredibly sophisticated medical means. Today we hardly cure more than we did 20 years ago and sometimes it is at great human cost.

This book is therefore a reflection, an eye-opener and a path to more humanism. Why would the body turn against itself ? Is the body you ? Where is the self ? Who is you ? The body as an extension of oneself ? Cancer as a cry of alarm to wake you up before moving into the great unknown.

To answer these multiple, difficult and mysterious questions which are humanistic, philosophical or even spiritual and transcendent, it will certainly be necessary to listen to oneself, then to the parts of oneself, thus to this very disturbing stranger, that our world calls Cancer !

So, this little book opens other possible paths: those of listening and asking some relevant questions about the initiate path that one enters with disease and specifically cancer - while asking these questions and listening to one or more answers, does not block the path to healing by using the Western therapeutic arsenal. This self-listening may help refine our scientific approaches and healing models while integrating the multiple methodologies of integrated therapies. Listening to the cancer entity may reveal, who knows, other approaches that we currently cannot even imagine possible.

In this book the diagnosis and forms of treatment are discussed taking the viewpoint of Cancer - barely representing the Western medical or scientific way but rather a holistic and humanistic and more spiritual approach not excluding, however, the angles of Western medicine. Various approaches will be discussed, the reflection of what since the end of the 1990s has been called "integrative approaches" !

This is of course NOT a scientific manual and is NOT meant to be medical. It is a book on a variety of approaches that punctuate the path of many people who have cancer. It must be remembered that according to national statistics of various Western countries, between 75 and 95% of patients who have cancer, will explore other approaches ranging from fasting therapy to raw diets, healers or other shamans of various cultures or countries. Remember also that the WHO (World Health Organization) lists many treatments that fall within traditional medicine and cannot be described as obsolete. Cultures and beliefs, from one country to another, are very different, and accordingly the therapeutic mode will be different.

Relapse, palliative or symptomatic care and end of life as well as death will be addressed since they are an integral part of the Cancer Path.

A wider outlook with spiritual and philosophical approaches will make this book a whole, and a guide in the multi-sense notion of this word.

Everything has been inspired by the author's approach through her own life path as an oncologist first in public hospitals, then private ones, as well as in her daily life as a private practitioner. Most thoughts will have been toyed with while sharing with the patient and / or their families.

Keep your mind open, and remember the iceberg, you only see the tip, as the 90% of it is submerged. Cancer and the human being are one and the same. So an open mind is the only possible motto because everything is always possible. It is up to you to maintain this link to the whole and the conviction that "all is possible".

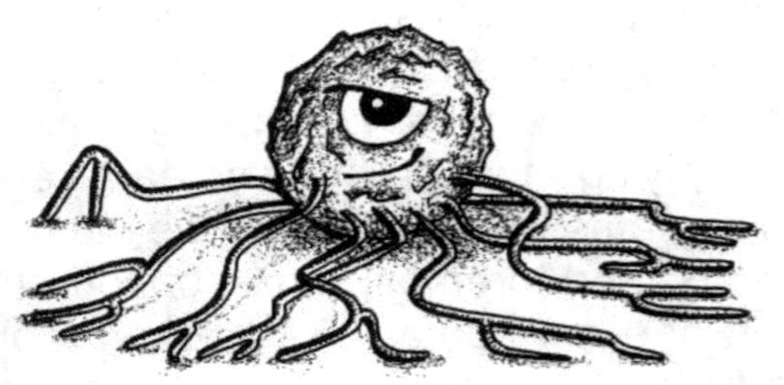

3 Cancer who are You ?

Oh, you mean Me ? I'm Me ! Well, well ! I'm surprised that I'm being called or listened to. It's pretty rare. Well, um, how shall I put it: I'm just me ! Multiple, alive, conscious, astonishing, fearful, whimsical, ill-mannered, yes, really bad, and so on and so forth.

I am also that part of you that dreams of breaking your chains, to say shit, I can't go on anymore, dreams of disobeying, of doing as you please, of dancing instead of complying - that part that screams and who screams wanting to stop the mess.
I am first and foremost a part of you and a part of every human being. Even a big part of you ... according to my or rather your aspirations and my, no, your dreams.

You were led to believe that I was only a group of cells that has gone crazy and immortal, do you believe that ? Oh, if you really knew who I am or who you are ! Oh dear, science I don't care much about its piffle, I'm much more than that .... I have existed since the dawn of time, I'm everywhere in the living world. I exist in the plant kingdom, in animals and I even exist in your head .... No, not in your brain but in your head, those crazy thoughts that go round and round and nearly make you mad ! Oh dear me you've been fed a very ugly image of Me.

Listen, I find that I am important and that I serve the cause .... I am useful ... I am a being in my own right but I can grow the way I wish and take up all the room. I can destroy what I find on my path to enlarge my private space ... when you need space, I answer and I take space. I also send emissaries anywhere I want ! These are little "Me's", but not totally Me anyway, and that makes Me resist everything you do and all your damn stuff to make Me die. By making Me die, I remind you that you are dying .... The more you try to eliminate Me, the more I gather strength ... Even if not always. You know, I can leave, sometimes. Your horrific poisons sometimes make me flee. They would scare anyone away, sooner or later.

I love this war and you know it serves My cause and your cause since you and Me, we are one and the same !

I'm giving you food for thought and when I speak it's not poppycock, wait and see, it's scholarly and I received it from much higher up, one night when I meditating on

Myself and my fate when you abused Me without listening to Me:

Cancer is a fractal of the One .... The One, trying to rearrange itself through the chaos to become the One again.

In addition, I also thought of Dion Fortune, a mystical woman and British occultist of the early 20th century who suggested that I was an entity with a powerful spiritual part. I confirm that to you, whether you like or not.

I have my life and my feelings and my spiritual guidance like you. I remind you that you are consciousness and that you are part of everything so I too am consciousness and I am also part of everything. I am.

3.1 Cancer, what's Your name ?

Aha! you humans love to name, it's crazy! I have a name and no name of course, but for you, it is good that I be named .... To talk about "my cancer" or the " crab " or "that thing" or the "thing " is so impersonal. What's worse is that you put me, as it were, out of you, as if I were not part of you.

I can call myself Mathew, Robert or Rachel or even William. You'll see, when you give me a name, it's the one which comes to you spontaneously. It'll make me damn less scary even if you hate me. Try to hate Robert in the same way as "my cancer": you'll really be astonished ! Funny how a name can change the whole outlook to something, but it does.

You will finally be surprised to find me closer and more "human", easier to listen to and get in touch with. Maybe one of these days, you'll be happy to have known Me, and you could love Me a little. More important is that My message will have percolated. You will begin to accept yourself and love yourself a wee bit.

I am a bit of truth: your truth.

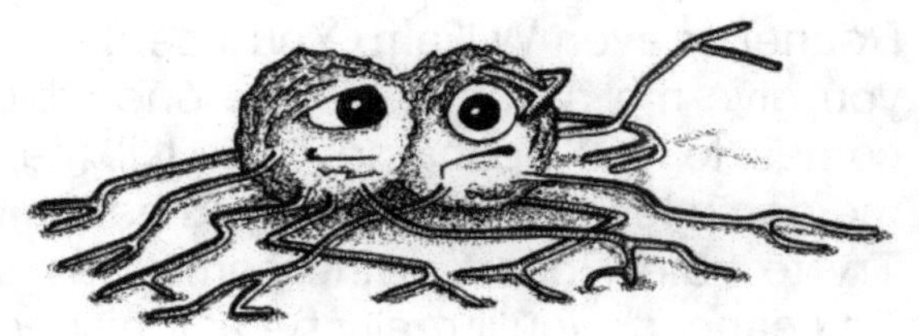

3.2 What does science say of You ?

Oh, scientists say a whole lot of things about Me. For them, I am only material. I do not exist as something else, as a proper entity. I am sometimes cells or genetic material of the name of DNA that has changed or mutated. These mutations and genetic changes are linked to fairly clear causes, from their point of view. These causes are mostly related to lifestyle and to the environment: because you've smoked too much, drunk booze or eaten too many additive's such as E 500 and so forth and so on. These mutations appear spontaneously following the ingestion of various "poisons" and they then lead the cell to go mad and to grow relentlessly and send out many emissaries !

I may be a bit of that and a bit of something else. Go and meet my friend Bruce Lipton (yes, yes I have friends too) if you do not want to be the victim of your genes, nor of your epigenetics and therefore of Me.
Besides, have the scientists, even once, taken the trouble to get in touch with Me? The fact is that no one can do without Me. I have become important, yes even very important. I love that, you may be sure !

Fear, that negative emotion that you hold deep within you ... do you know about that, are you conscious ? Go and explore those molecules of emotions, and their amazing woman scientist Candace Pert. The more you are afraid, the more I love! Fear has a smell, a feeling maybe even a color, have you ever thought of that ? It develops transmitters deep inside you. This fear can change your cells, your internal biotope. Have a look at the meaning of biotope.
Must I remind you that your cells are bathing galore in this biotope called fundamental substance.

You know, I am very sensitive and I also react a great deal to negative stimuli that each human holds within himself. You hold a rather nasty view of Me and of yourself, but like you, I can be nice and helpful or even be innocuous or terrible, or prickly, or even be a screamer or a murderer ...like you. You can disappear from the face of the earth in a few weeks! I have many, many things to tell you about you ! I am amazing. And I am aware of that ! Are you ?

Every time you can't go on anymore I come on the back stage, a little ... your internal moods change and I feel it. When you get pissed off by saying that you can't live like this anymore and so on, I peep in and I start wondering if the time has come to help you in your process of change, to open up and to listen to yourself perhaps? I've been listening to you since day one as I am a part of you. I'm a sort of guardian maybe ?

I've always wondered why you don't listen and this is what made you call Me. When I arrive it is often to sweep everything widely away ... and in addition you hate Me .... do you not know that I'm a part of you ... maybe you've forgotten ? that I am also in you because you are also this body, this spirit and this soul. Sometimes I am very sad that you don't want Me. I ask of you to at least inquire about Me, please ! For and by the love of you, for the sake of who you are. Yes, I do astound you ! Have you once taken the time to ask Me what I am doing here ?

4 Cancer, how dare You knock on my
   door ?

Aha ! You make me laugh ! Maybe you
needed Me ?.... Might you have called Me
to get you out of a grizzly situation ? .... to
give you some time for reflection and
change. Call me loudly enough and I'm
here, I'm your man ! Oh, you know maybe
that you're not very aware of what you do
or of your powers ... You call and I come,
it's not to hurt you ... I don't want to do
that! I come to help in the process of
departure or transformation, or help you
to leave a job that you hate, or to get away
from a woman or a man that you abhor or
to open you up to another place, or
something else or another way of doing
or seeing things. I'm your wake up call.

It's possible that long before you came
into this life, before you were born, you
chose, (not you here and now, but a part
of you, your soul or your spiritual
substance   pre-incarnation),   this
experience to live. This experience was
going to help to know You, to remember
who You are or where You come from ...
or to experiment or to help others to
experiment or even to allow you to leave
this earth to join your loved one's on the
other side. I also serve as a way out !
Have you thought of the exit door - you

have sometimes really called for it !
Please do your research on death and
even more so on your death, you need to.
I seriously advise you.

Sometimes, I am the result of a family
history. You are like your mother and your
grandmother before you. Maybe I am a
memory of a distant grandmother, or
great grandmother who is still suffering.
Did you know that one could still suffer
many centuries later ? Now that opens up
a revealing thought, doesn't it ?

Did you ever imagine that I could come
from somewhere else, or from before
your life started ? That you're also the
human result of a past, or of some human
history or other. Mind-boggling, isn't it ?
and I'm not talking about genetic history;
But your genes are also your past, your
history, your story. Go and read about
genealogy. There are many books on the
subject. Do a family constellation, in
accordance with Bert Hellinger or in a
similar line of thought. Most interesting.
You are your past, you are your grandma
and so on and so forth.

Ask questions if there is still living
"memory": a grandmother, even better, a
great-grandmother or elderly people who
might remember. Again, you will learn a

whole lot of things. That your father is your grandfather or a German soldier and things like that. Family secrets, in the human race, are always of a similar nature, where shame and guilt are present. They're always about death, sex, money or madness. However, all this you know in the depths of your substance.

There is always a reason for things being the way they are. It's up to you to know yourself and to know this part of you that is in pain, to know your family history or your origins or even the lack of history and of origin.
Everything has a sense, and I assure you that if there is not, there is a reason to worry. Albert Einstein, a great thinker, said: "In appearance life has no meaning, and yet it is impossible that it hasn't got one".
I remind you once again that it's all about you. Go and ponder on the meaning of your life.

4.1 Are You a punishment ?

Oh crumbs, why would I be a punishment? Who put that idea into your head or into your heart ? Why should you be punished and if so by whom or by what ? Have you done something so awful ? And who decides what is awful or not ?!? Your question offends me, upsets me and surprises me, but finally I like it when you question me. It's the proof that you're thinking and changing, and that you're daring to open to your own light a little more.

Ah ! So you thought then that I'm a divine punishment for having smoked, drunk or raped. Even today a lady, who's otherwise very enlightened, asked Clare, whether the return of her lymphoma was a punishment for something she had done, but she did not figure out what. Beliefs in punishment are strongly embedded in your unconscious. Hmmm... your god is really angry and petty. The idea of an angry god is well anchored in the Judeo-Christian history and has been established for about 4000 years. And it's those 4000 years of hegemony of this god and beliefs around him that still play on your unconscious mind. This way of thinking doesn't disappear so easily from our collective fields. Remember to revisit

your beliefs and see if they're really yours or whether they belong to others !
Tell me, who runs your life ? Is it you or the belief system belonging to others ? Is it what you have been brought up on ? Is there an outside god ? Or are you an entity and a spark of the divine ?
If you believe in a hell fire is that not your internal reality ? Must you be punished for being alive ? Do you really think you learn your lesson by being punished ? What is punishment, other than your feelings of guilt, listening to a reference outside of yourself. Maybe to smoke, to drink or to rape isn't of a good idea, but does it mean that you need to punish yourself and to beat yourself because of that....

To dare say out loud what some people think deep inside, may also be one of my roles !

Well, no, I am neither a punishment nor anything else. I am a reflection of your beliefs. If you think you should be punished then you will be punished; if you think you have to pay for a possible act, then you will be. I encourage you, on my arrival, to begin to revisit your belief system about yourself and who you are. Indeed Joan of Arc was burned at the stake, on the belief that she was possessed ... a belief, no more no less.

4.2 Hey, Cancer, could I've avoided You?

O heavens !, it's too late to ask such a question ! You called me, and I arrived, I sometimes roamed a little or sometimes I came galloping and now you will have to make do with my presence. Are you angry ? furious ? Sad ? Do you accuse your neighbour, your wife, your job: hold on, just be honest with yourself. You could've changed jobs, left your wife or moved house ... With Me, you'll have to listen to Me: yes, you can cut Me, burn Me, poison Me. I may leave of course, only to come back, better than before, closer, bigger, greater, changed in other words with Me it's another story, and the more you're afraid…. I love that, and the more you're afraid, the stronger I get. I feed on you and your locked up emotions. Give me a little of your time and your openness and you will understand why I am here. Perhaps we can then negotiate, reach a compromise, better still a consensus !!

What do you risk by listening to Me ? In my humble opinion not much, as I'm already there. At best change the situation; at worst accept it and move on. I just want to tell you. Why did you wait so long ? Did you not see the warning signs, the absolute necessity to listen to yourself and to change ?..... Anyway, I encourage you to pull up your socks and get going along the road again, it's never too late. You are actually so powerful, beyond all that you believe ! Listen to me and above all, listen to yourself.

4.3 The Truth

I hear the word truth, what is the truth ?
Who has the truth ?

What is the truth anyway and who holds
the truth ? Why should I listen to You ?
But crumbs, because I'm you. You're
right, you know how to lie to yourself, to
hide your head in the sand, pretend, but
deep down inside, when you really think
about it, you know, you really know. It's
there your truth: well hidden in the depth
of you, under the pile of "false
everything's", the inculcated which is so
perverse, the non-listening and the
unsaid, the non-daring.
Decide to listen to yourself and stop being
scared. Scared of what ? Of Me ? No of
you and your truth.
Go and look it in the face !
Do you want to be My victim ? Oh yes !
you know for yourself. You know if you
take the trouble to listen. Have you often
listened to yourself ? The truth is that you
let others decide for you, you've been
doing it throughout your life. You've quite
simply given up your power and in
addition, you firmly believe that it's the
others who know. Learn to distinguish
between information and knowledge.

Learn to dare, listen to yourself without letting anyone stop you. It's all about learning, I concede but I encourage you to start, and straight away. Take small steps, it's always easier. Do you really like the job where you work ? Or going to your mother-in-law's house for Sunday lunch ? I 'm not saying you should not go but think about it, take the time to observe, to observe yourself, to ask yourself one or two questions: maybe you haven't got the answers or maybe you have them but you do not even dare to look at them. Look inside yourself and observe again and again, breathe and take time.

Why are you always running ? Where are you running to ? And to what ? Have you ever realized that you are running towards your own death, imagining that you might escape it ?.... I tell you, this is the only thing we can all be sure about. Death is part of life, but it is also life.

4.4 Have You given me warning signs ?
    What do You have to say to me ?

Of course ! it is extremely rare that I come to you out of the blue.
When you asked for a solution to do with leaving your husband and you didn't dare? Or, with leaving a job where you were a slave, or were being bullied. After your second burn-out, you needed something strong to stop you from going back to that "mine" that was gradually killing you. You see when I arrive it is often with the great melodrama and noise! It's never easy when I'm here.
Remember when, after your wife was unfaithful, you started bleeding from the rectum: I was getting ready to come. Fortunately you took things in hand just in time, and you left the situation. There, the mix between your awareness, your actions and the surgeon brought about a direct healing. Surgery is sometimes easier than trying to make the "thing" go away through your thought process and your intention ! Even if theoretically it is quite possible.
But surgery alone may not be the answer. And I'm not talking about anything else but listening to me or rather to you.

I often come to save you, and help you get out of a bad situation: but at what a price !

Take your life in hand as soon as possible and before my arrival, please ! In this I am your friend. I suggest you change: turn off the TV and go out and enjoy nature, eat less and healthier, move, meditate, breathe and listen and create. Create a better life for yourself. Spend less time and money on futilities ! that way you can earn less money and therefore work less. Your overall balance will improve.

These are of course, only suggestions but, at least ask yourself some questions and who knows, you'll maybe get some answers.

5 Cancer, what am I going to do with
  You ?

Listen to Me, but especially, and above all, listen to you, no more, no less: a deep profound existential listening.

A new set of steps for you ! I will try to guide you and show you a different path. A new existence and way of life. I encourage you to stick to it, body and soul. Seek new ways of doing things, learn to use your discernment, open up, grope, observe what's right inside you and in depth. This is certainly not the easiest way, but you are free to do as you wish !

You will need people around you: ask for various opinions, maybe 2 or 3. When you have found some good people, say doctors or therapists to help you, you will have your magic circle. Expand it as you wish but be careful, avoid losing yourself. Take time, on a daily basis to refocus and listen to you. Your "You" time. And know that you need it, and that furthermore, you're entitled to it.

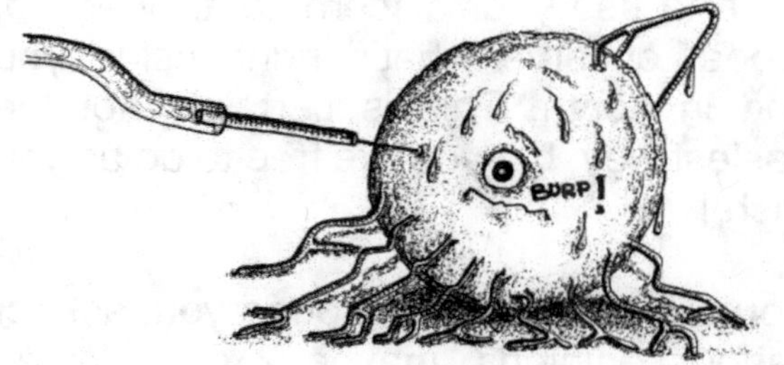
BURP!

5.1 What are the heavy treatments to
       knock You out ?

So, when you have to do to with Me, you
will also have to do with countless doctors
and other professionals who revolve
around Me ! Now, you're considered a
really sick person, not an impostor. You
have a real illness, Me ! You are taken
seriously, yes, very seriously and they will
attempt to take care of Me, not of you, not
necessarily of either of us in fact, but of
that entity called cancer, the physical Me,
which is created by your doctors and
other scientists. And it's all very serious
.... consultations, examinations, over and
over. I will be viewed from all angles as a
rare beast. Needles will be inserted inside
you, to know the color of my eyes, or my
skin. A very serious evaluation will be
made of Me. Well, I can tell you right now
it's only a tiny portion of Me, but they think
they know.

Depending on which "box" they put Me in,
you will be enlisted in a protocol. There
are many serious protocols ! There are
the ... International, the French, the
American, the British, even the European
etc. and the names of these protocols are
rather weird like ECOG, ESTRO, MRC,
SAKK, ASTRO followed by numbers etc.
etc. And there you have it ! A computer

may even choose your path. It takes quite a crack brain, to try to understand who, where and what are the truths. It's an extremely difficult maze.
And you and I, we hear all this and not sure that we understand neither one or the other.

If you have a doctor, an oncologist, who's slightly more enlightened, he or she may offer you a potpourri of his or her experience, something more personal maybe ... but always combining their winning team, the gold standard: surgery, radiation or drugs. The drugs are what they prefer: there will be some that are red and fluorescent, some that don't stand even the smallest amount of light, and so on and so forth. You will be sick, maybe you'll through up or you'll lose your hair or your nails, you'll be really ill, pale, anemic, tired, maybe very tired. And besides there's this never ending merry go round: this hellish rhythm, every week, every two weeks or even three, and the damn cycle of their holy protocols. The more they are toxic for your life, the more the medical human seems to think that it'll be effective. Me, from My point of view, that of My humble self, I am not so sure, but the studies, yes those famous studies and protocols, seem to prove it, unless ....

Difficult to find one's way through this labyrinth of medical battles. For the time being, that is now, it's the golden way to get rid of Me and sometimes your life too but it would seem that I'm exaggerating. What do you think ?

From time to time, I just disappear: Oh just a wee bit; I pretend to leave through the scalpel of the handsome surgeon. It's awesome and scary at the same time. They are always masculine and good looking and I love them as feminine and softer, they often have more sensitivity and take you, more into account. Do you know that it is rare that surgery really does remove me ? Am I really in your body ? They cut Me out and they say Hooray we took it all out, it's wonderful but, the famous "but" ...
Then, they go on to say: well you may need .... some chemotherapy or radiotherapy, you know, it's just in case. I say just in case of what ? Either I am gone, or I am here, but I am not of a "just in case" ! besides I do not like this way of speaking to you and to Me. You can't address us both in such an aloof manner.

Well, in some contexts they definitely liquidate me. I then stay in a quiet, hiding place and I watch. I wonder if they really had me, and what part of Me they have stunned ... because I can stay a long, long time waiting. Did you know this: it seems that if every male lived up to a hundred years there would be cells of Me in his prostate ... yes ... these are autopsy results ... and, listen, the best of all this: they did not die because of Me !

In human time, I can stay dormant maybe 25-30 years and surreptitiously, I reappear. Sometimes in the same place but more often in a place that suits Me and in line with our mutual history: you are sad and can't take it anymore, I migrate into your lungs, you're completely entangled, I go to your brain, where there is rage and anger and I'm into your liver. If you are really at a loss, then I go everywhere, all over your structure. It's just to help you, I assure you, I am you and you are Me. Funny equation anyway! Lay this equation down and you'll understand, it's mathematical !

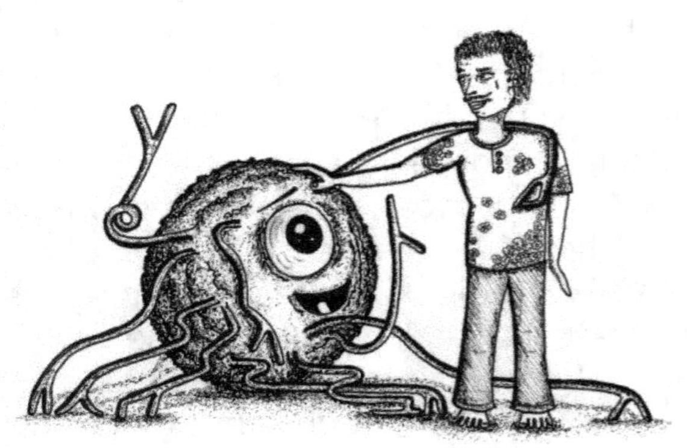

5.2 What are the soft options for getting
    rid of You ?

Ah !! know yourself, all the answers are within. Start listening, again and again.

First and foremost, is to listen to your own power within. Yes, listen to you ! Elementary, really ! How long is it since you listened to you ? Be honest. In My opinion, it's been a very long time. So start by listening to yourself and take a few moments to refocus. Please avoid letting yourself be embarked by the outside world and the system and even more so by fear: this system wants everything fast, fast, fast ! You'll see that when I arrive in your life everything goes helter-skelter as if we were at the end of time. Think about this ! I've been here for a while and I've been waiting for this moment with impatience and delight when at last you have realized my existence, my presence. Doctors rob you of this exchange, this precious moment, by accelerating everything to prevent you from taking your life into your own hands! In My opinion they steal your life, can you see that ?!

You see, Cancer, that's Me in this case, is in your mind. It is there first. I hardly got there overnight: I'm not the spontaneous kind. I've been called in, I think I'm late but at a given time I decide or rather you decide that I will come into your life, to help you move forward ! So I'm in your mind before being in your body and there's no sense in asking why or how. I'm in you and you will have to change your mind to change your body.

And to change your mind, it will be useful to look at your life with honesty: all aspects of your life: from A to Z. If you start from the assumption that what you created you can undo, you can change anything ! It's not so clear, of course, in your black or white thought system.
You can fight me. You'll get tired at that game: exhaustion is at the end of that road. You must take hold of your life. It's YOU who must be in the driver's seat, no one can lead your life for you and yet that's what happens implicitly when you let others decide for you.

So come with Me and listen to Me. Take control of your life and look at all portions of it. Make quick changes but in-depth ones. Support your body but remember that you are not your body. Your body is your earthly vehicle for a given time. A vehicle, neither more nor less, even if taking care of it is, certainly, a good thing.

"No one knows the day or hour when these things will happen". This old biblical adage is spot on from my point of view !

So, start by listening to yourself, learn to meditate. Stop running around like a headless chicken, after Prada shoes or your next holidays in the Caribbeans or even, how you're going to pay the bills at the end of the month. Look at all sections of your life: your diet, your sleep, the number of hours you spend looking at television or sitting in front of your computer. When did you last observe nature ? Stroke the cat ? How do you feel? Do you even feel ?

When you have observed your life a little, start bringing about changes and quickly. Do not let laziness overtake you ... go on, it takes courage to change a life of habits and particularly unhealthy habits.
Look at your relationships, there too, start the spring-cleaning. Those that bother you most, do they prevent you from evolving, from being more authentic and true to yourself ? Get rid of them or change them.

All along this path, you can, of course, combine all the options, but take care to clarify your inner motives and your beliefs about this or that.

Well then, what are the soft options to make Me clear out ? You see, there too, you will find everything and the contrary. What I can tell you is that all ways of boosting your immune system, will help you live your life. But you must want to *live* life. And remember that your conscious thought is only a tiny part of who you are, even a microscopic part: often you will say yes, I want to live but deep inside, you do not know whether you do or not, because life on earth isn't easy. Again, find someone to help you, but most of all, learn to know yourself. If I am here, there is a reason even if you can't see it !

When you have got onto your path, start by changing one thing, yes only one thing: help your body, of course, if not you won't be alive any more. Above all, support your immune system, but remember, it all starts in the mind so begin to change your way of thinking.

If you have pain take care of it. Look at this from all points of view and especially try to listen to what it is trying to say to you. If it is too strong, take some pills or other medication. You can take methadone (see Dr. Claudia Friesen, ULM university) or cannabis - both are amazing ! Oh no, it's not only for those people whom you categorize too quickly as junkies or addicts. Beware of judgments, they can boomerang back on you. Remember, what you think is what you are !!

Reach into your internal realm and also look at your external: both have amazing effects as anti Me. Well, I'll tell you they're not really against Me, they just allow you to take back a piece of your own power. Remember that it is first of all in your power and not to swallow X, Y or Z without thought as medication. Me, I am well beyond that sort of stupidity. I am very clever, brilliant in fact !

There is no big or small miracle says the book of Helen Schucman and William Thetford, "A Course in Miracles". You can also get interested in this type of reading that opens your mind towards consciousness and renewal, a new form of spirituality, coming from other planes of existence.

Take a look at vitamin C and its champion scientist Linus Pauling, Nobel Prizewinner. There are many scientific studies, even if not "mainstream", on its powerful role, for your immune system. The best way to take it is directly through infusion into your veins: doses ranging from a few grams to over 100g. The risks are low and the benefits great. Be careful if you take it by mouth to use buffered capsules or a liposomal preparation, otherwise beware of diarrhea !

Another medical approach to which you may give some thought is that of Rudolf Steiner and the Anthroposophists. The approach is wide, holistic and interesting, but I encourage you to leave the dogmas aside, it's not because the approach is global that it's good for you. Always be discerning even if that's something new to you and apply this advice to everything and to all parts of your life. But do remember that strangely enough, discernment changes with belief.
The anthroposophists have some very interesting and trusted products to help you overcome Me, without doing you too much harm. The doctors of the allopathic world will tell you that they are potions, but have they looked at theirs ? They are also potions, but with familiar names and crazy prices ! But they are potions all the same. There are competing doctrines, of course, frequently not even remotely overlapping.

The famous fermented mistletoe, or Iscador, from the anthroposophical compendium is amongst these amazing forms of treatment. It's a real treatment, I assure you and you'll see, it won't hurt you and means I will take up a little less room.

Finally even if it makes me decamp, I like this treatment because I leave of my own free will. And you know, there is even science behind it, yes your sacred science, the living God. You make me laugh with your science stuff ! Maybe it reassures you that God is with you even if you reject this idea per se, it is still deeply ingrained in your genes and in your deep unconscious beliefs. Well I tell you that it is in all things even in Me. It makes you shudder, so shudder and ask yourself a few more questions, deeper and more philosophical ones.

Turmeric is also an interesting addition, deserving of being integrated into your potential therapeutic arsenal. It has many virtues widely used in Ayurveda medicine.

Vitamin B17, or Laetrile, is not recognized by conventional medicine. Studies are controversial, and yet the famous FDA, the American control organ for medication, has removed it completely from the market by stipulating that it is dangerous. But, I encourage you to take a look. As for the notion of its being dangerous: Life is dangerous and chemotherapy too, but are they illegal ? The controversy comes from the FDA's assertion that it has no positive effects whereas some studies, show very clear beneficial effects. I can't give you my clear opinion, explore, just be very careful over listening to your inner being, you will know if it's right or not. Far from me to say that dangerous is good. It depends on what is meant by dangerous !

The cures of Rudolph Breuss, Max Gerson, Catherine Kousmine, and Hulda Clarke are all different approaches and in some cases have produced spectacular results, but they are all only recipes. I encourage you to go further than a recipe and find your own way or your own path.

Healers such as John of God, the Brazilian, Alex Orbito, the Filipino, Alexandre Jodorowsky and his psycho magic in his Parisian café-theatre, Lourdes with its St Bernadette and its holy water well or Our Lady of Fatima in Portugal have both adepts and detractors: here too there have been some surprising cures and of course some nil results, this being seen through the lenses of the left brain and Western attitudes. Any method practiced with faith and intention can defy the laws of Newtonian science, and will go through other more quantum ways. If the presupposition is that everything is possible, then logically everything will become possible. Do the experimentation for yourself.

Carl Simonton, who is at the origin of The Simonton cancer centers around the world, in his book "An Adventure of Healing" reports very clearly the effect of beliefs on our healing. The importance therefore remains to deal with your beliefs. If you think you can heal by taking Lourdes water then it becomes possible while for another, you are a moron to have even thought about it. Therefore it is you, who defines what's possible. On the other hand, if you adhere to the facts that the medical science and its limited point of view tells you, you cut yourself off from all these other possibilities. The placebo effect and its opposite, the nocebo effect have an important place in any cure. It can represent up to 70% of the result.

You make me laugh just a bit. You humans think that a simple molecule will save you: save what ? Let me ask ?

Rid you of Me ? You make Me laugh
because, I'm you.

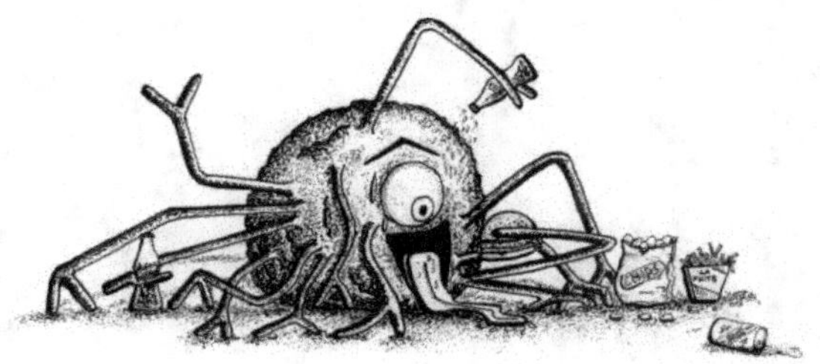

5.3 What are Your thoughts on food ?

Food, is it a hobby of yours ? Do you want: only fresh food, or the Paleolithic, or the vegan, the gluten-free, the sugar-free and ketogenic, and so on and so forth.
Food is a difficult subject. Beliefs and dogmas abound. The real knowledge about this subject, is hard to find. You will find studies of all sorts, with everything and the contrary.

Food ? Important or not ? I do not know if I can really answer you.
Some humans, the most daring and avant-garde, perhaps, say that it is a medicine in its own right.
From my point of view, I totally agree ! Food, the outlook on food, which is even more important, plays a fundamental role in My life and in yours.
Have you looked at your food ? What is it for you ? How are you eating ? Or what are you eating ? How does your body react to your way of eating food ? Do you need this or that ? What's good for you ? Do you even know what's in the dish you are eating ? Or where do the eggs or the beans, that you put in your shopping cart, come from ? Is the chicken happy or not?

Does your pig have to travel for hours, and in what condition, before being slaughtered ? "Tell me what you eat, I'll tell you whom you are" said Anthelme Brillat-Savarin, the famous French cook. Or again, this old Maghrebi proverb of the years 1855: "The less man eats, the more his heart fills with light". And these saying are as old as the hills !

Eating is a big and complex subject. Go, dig, read, listen to your body and your senses, your internal guidance, and if you do not know how to do it, try to learn. Coca cola, ketchup and chips are they really good for you ? On the other hand, remember that nothing is ever completely good or completely bad: it depends on the circumstances and also on the outlook and belief's you have. There is food for thought, I admit. Besides, should we be perfect ? and who lays down the criteria of this perfection.

Non-eating also has its followers ... (see Thierry Lestrade on the therapeutic fast and its uses) and the followers of "prana", nourished by light, astonishing, aren't they ? Feeding with light exists and not only among gurus and yogis of the East.

I also remind you that all life comes from a conjunction of multiple factors and one of those is water. Take care of the water, drink enough water, bless your water to improve its vibration. One of the possible scientific explanations on the miracles of Lourdes would be that the water from its source would have a very high vibratory rate linked to an unknown... The vibratory rate is important since it will allow a change of state. Think about all this and please take care of yourself and the water. You are, one and the other important ! Besides, you are water !

As part of your body, I need you to nourish Me and bring me food, no more and no less. I (Rachel, William or even Mathew) can come in spite of your healthy and organic food, your failures or your diets, your fasting and your meditations, your yoga or your various techniques of listening to yourself. Well, once I'm here, change something, it's certainly a method, to help Me or rather to help you, it's rather to help you !
I'm not sure that I need help, I have a lot of resources !!

Try, but above all, to learn to really listen to yourself. Look at your beliefs and your habits, your how's and your why's. You will learn about yourself. Decrease the too much or increase the not enough. Take a look at your thoughts and their visions of lack or excess ! Beliefs all come from there ... Or almost. They start in your head or rather in your mind.

5.4 Is my life style important ?

Way of life is a massive part of your life. It is by definition on planet earth a major programming system. It will depend on: where you were born, and in what thought or religious system you were brought up. Your psychic and emotional way of being and the state of the earth where you are living. If you live on the edge of the ocean or in a city slum, the data will be different.

Your way of life contributes to your life. It certainly generates lots of beliefs. Read, listen, choose within the limits of your possibilities and especially expand your possibilities! Use your discernment and inner skills, and expand your skills and beliefs as well as your discernment. And remember that if you know that something is harmful for you, you should do your best to change it.

It is fairly clear that smoking is harmful to your health, but it will depend on many other factors. If you smoke 5 cigarettes/day or if you smoke 3 packs/day without any thought, the result on your health will obviously be different. Everything is a matter of degree and balance. The roads of excess never seem good !

Have you thought of how you feel when you smoke three packets of cigarettes a day or drink 15 whiskeys ? Of course I'll let you answer according to your own vision and especially, your own feelings. Why do you need 15 glasses of whiskey a day ? The question may be there. And I'm not asking you to stop but just to become aware ! Are you, or should you be the master of your life ?! No ? The awareness will be your answer, then you will decide what action is needed to effect the change.

Having fun, taking time to laugh, listening to music or dancing and sharing, sharing a lot with those who are good for you is a MUST. Creating through art, music, poetry, sculpture, drawing will help you and your cells. Remember molecules of emotions!

Eating in good company, drinking a good tea or even a small glass of port, in moderation but please learn how to taste. There is no need for passionate desires to have fun! A walk in the forest or at the water's edge can be a mystical moment of exaltation. Enjoy life. And try to start before my arrival, it would be better.

5.5 Listening to yourself, to Me and to your body

First let Me remind you that you are NOT a body. Your body is your earthly vehicle for this life. It is, of course, part of you for a given time when you are here on earth. I also remind you that there are a multitude of bodies of all kinds, that you do not even know exist. These bodies are around you like a second skin. So maybe it would be good to talk about the physical body, the one made of what you call matter. This body is an extension of everything that animates you. It is the visible part of the iceberg. Even if this surprises you, I am only partially in your body! When I come back on stage, things have already happened in your mind. In a way, I'm like the tip of the iceberg. Astonishing isn't it ?

So, while you can take good care of your body, it may well be illusory. You will have to take care of the entirety of who you are, including your embodied plane. When your body screams, it is because you too are screaming your head off. The misfortune is that nobody hears you! Well that's not quite true in fact, since I'm waiting patiently to bring you my help. The most dramatic part in all this, is that

you don't want my help, not in the least !
Yet.

I suggest you listen to you, learn how and learn fast. Be like Me, if you must: ill-mannered, screaming, angry, yelling and so on. You can at least free yourself from some strong and toxic emotions that you have accumulated. Guess where? In your body! Oh yes .... I'm a great teacher!

So, your first job is to go inwards and listen to you, and do it quickly. Your time is running out. Besides, it always has been. Let me remind you that no one knows either the day or the hour, and when I arrive it is perhaps a little sooner than you had imagined in your all sufficient power.
Your body is a sensor and an amazing antenna. It informs you over and over at any and all times. It's phenomenally sensitive.

It is also, by default, a rubbish bin and you know what happens when you don't empty the trash ? Take a look at the Diogenes syndrome on your tablet or laptop please. You're going to be shocked and horrified and say "That's not me" but who knows maybe it is !

Now let's talk about your I-pad, or your I-Phone or your I-something else. Do you have any idea what these objects can do to your bodies ? Don't you call them smart phones or similar ? They are smart, they're too captivating, maybe too smart and too captivating. Did you know that they have a toxicity which has not yet been completely elucidated, the lobbies are so strong and so important. The international study "Mobi-kids" currently underway, proposes a code of use for this telephony, taking into account the principle of precaution. The precautionary principle is good to my mind, I always encourage an enlightened vision. So, get enlightened and remember to feel, and to go within yourself, asking three and a half questions.

5.6 What about emotions ?

Lise Bourbeau, a Canadian best-selling author, well known for her various books on listening to one's self and to one body, writes about 5 major and fundamental wounds. Those deep and existential wounds that condition the life of each individual from his conception to recovery or death!

Rejection, abandonment, humiliation, betrayal and injustice: five fundamental injuries that cause our ills, whether physical, emotional or mental.
Who hasn't tried to please no matter what? Who let himself become the shadow or the puppet of his mother or father.

Your emotions, and especially those you are not proud of, have been buried deep inside of you and relegated to the bottom and the darkest part of you. Injury after injury, time takes its toll, and of course Me. Some useful readings are listed below.

Cancer is a fractal of the One ... The One trying to rearrange itself through chaos to become One again.

Think about it when nothing goes well. Have you forgotten that you are you, in you and in all ? So, you are all.

When a parent said certain things to you, was that you, were you being told obliquely that you had to grow up to become extraordinary, perfect, heroic, or insignificant, unobtrusive ??

You forgot simply to be yourself. You didn't dare be you. You simply forgot to live, to laugh, to cry or scream. The guilt of simply existing and not being what someone else wanted you to be, but just be you.

5.7 Is there a place for guides or guardian
     angels ?

Believe it or not, I'm a guide, had you
thought about that ? I am also guided and
I have a mentor, and you ?
My guide and mentor is called "Diabé",
funny name really, but it seems that it's
his name and it means the male wolf. He
whispered it in my right ear, at midnight
on a full moon. Wolves are like that!
Do you have a guide ? Clare's guide is
Orpheus, do you know him ? Do you
believe in such things ?.
Do you know Bashar or Abraham Hicks ?
They are also guides and they speak
through quite serious people. Dammit, if
your sacrosanct science heard me ! I
shudder at the thought. Anything new
must first exist in the mind. So, let's listen
to spirit. Keep your critical mind and your
discernment. What is crazy for some is
innovative for the others and a new reality
for the followers on. Think of Galileo, he
was almost burnt at the stake for saying
that the earth was round !

Does it seem funny to you that I'm
guided? but yes, I'm guided too. You are
too ? Take some time to listen and ask for
your guide's name. It will just come to
you, on the spur of the moment or out of
the blue.

Everywhere, in your daily life, you receive multiple signs of guidance, but in general, you have your nose down on the grindstone and you can't even get the first inkling! Do take the time to breathe, to feel and to watch and you will see the signs are everywhere. Guidance is in everything. As for guardian angels or other guides they are everywhere too. Einstein said that "Coincidence is God's way of remaining anonymous". Just think of that! What is chance or coincidence ? What is it or who is God ? No, I'm not talking about that angry and bearded guy on his cloud, that of your old book. That one is obsolete. No, look into you ? What is your resemblance with say: an ant or a lizard, or a cloud ? Ask yourself three and a half questions ... Important the half, do you know why ?

Perhaps because you can formulate the next half .... Go on! Learn to observe and reflect, to have a critical look at things and what is. Learn to discern, to dare to see things differently, to question, without losing yourself in doubt. Just dare... shake the pillars of certainty, of your certainty. Are you sure that this or that person is good for you ? Where are your childlike eyes ? And the ability to say NO, I don't want, above all I just can't. Learn to question by going into yourself and if, your guardian angel was no more than a part of you ? Have you thought about that? And what an incredible part, omniscient and highly powerful.

By changing your point of view and really listening to you, you are already going to change yourself. By changing yourself, you will of course change everything.
And how ? Through the morphogenetic fields. You and the other become one. So, when you change, you change the other too. There's an interesting guy, much discredited of course, but he dares to state his truth. Yes, these are morphogenetic fields, those of Sheldrake but also a bit like Jung. These explain that when a mouse finds its way in a labyrinth in Tokyo another mouse in a similar labyrinth, but in Panama also finds its way. This is of course without visual contact and conscious knowledge of one another. The information passed between the two mice as if by magic. Does the communication move through other fields? For your great-grandmother, the phone would have been pure magic, and yet you know it's not. Sheldrake's fields are like this, he is just a little avant-garde!

Our friend Carl Gustave Jung would have spoken of collective unconscious, which is also a sort of field. Had you heard of

that before ? And if not go and read a little
bit about it.

6 And when You come back ?

Oh dear ! Listen, I love and I love you more than anything else since I am an integral part of you. I can come back, here or elsewhere within your bodily system. I love to gain space when you don't listen. I want you to listen to Me, want you to take Me into account, seriously, but at least have you listened to Me. Far too often you lose yourself, for all kinds of reasons. You will tell Me that they are of course all good but they are not necessarily good for you. Have you forgotten your childhood dreams ? Have you lost that faculty to marvel ? To take the path so dear to your heart ? But no, you go back into the conditioning of your parents, grandparents or ancestors before you. It's the path of "you can't" "you don't", "you do not have the right to" "you're naughty" or "your grandfather would never have allowed that". And so on and from year to year, you lock yourself in. You lock up your light, your desires, your creativity and your dreams... until the day I arrive. And, as if in a flash, you wake up and you cry, Oh NO ! Suddenly, life is worth living and there you are, ready for a few moments, to listen to YOU - until you fall back into the groove, that of leaving your power to others. But please don't go fighting for

your life, by only ingesting chemicals or drugs. You'll forget yourself again in that fight ... and I'll come back and say "listen to Me" or "listen to you" because you and I are the same!
Life is very difficult - and so is the human mind!

7 When I win the game, what do You
  do ?

When you win, it's ok ! I simply retire and let you get on with your life. I stay aware and observe from My pedestal elsewhere. I see that you often ruin the life that you wanted so much, but that is your problem. Did you really want this life?

I'm a good loser or maybe you're a good winner ... anyway, it must be that way. I take French leave in a certain way. Maybe I'll come back, maybe not. We'll see. It's rather mysterious. I'm not into all the secrets. There are many more evolved beings above Me. What do you think? that you are alone in the universe? that there is only one universe. Hey-No ! There are multiverse, and "multi infinite". Put all this into perspective, I beg of you.

7.1 What does winning really mean ?

A very big dilemma is that of winning. What does it really mean, to win ?

With Me, you will win a challenge, a tortuous road, a lot of adventure, sensations and strong emotions.

I need you to win. So, I too, will feel that I have won in my role as a guide. A teacher is inseparable from a pupil. That's logic in a team. I'm a little of that for you. Sometimes you are the master, sometimes it's Me. It's finally not more important than that ? Unless you think differently ?

I'll let you meditate and be judge, of course.

8 Can I live with You ?

Of course, you can live with Me: we must find a common ground no more no less. But it may not be easy. I am far from convenient and easy going.

You know, science will tell you that 50% of Georges and other forms of Me, will be permanently destroyed by their treatments. But listen, I claim that they are not always spot on. They forget the people who do less well or even catastrophically after their "shock" treatments. So, then there's bias in their studies in one way or another, consciously or not, a bias brought in all too easily. And I'm not talking about fake studies or unrealistic treatments. Ask Clare, she knows a lot. We must walk together for a time and for the best and sometimes for the worst. I love to quibble, and make dirty jokes: that's altogether Me!

It is therefore difficult to put all these people and all these " Me's " in a meaningful study that demonstrates with an exact and mathematical certainty, a result about humans. Well, that's the way I see things.

So, the other 50% will die with Me on board. For a good 1/4 of them, we will walk together for many years. We must, by default, cooperate a little or even ideally find a degree of consensus ! You see, I can be a friend ... or at least a little less of an enemy !!

My behavior is far from simple. I do not like to say who I am or where I am, let alone talk about My case. Unveil my secrets, it's not easy for Me. Am I a little like you ? When you deceived your wife and you kept it deep inside, when you stole in the locker room or when you planned to kill your father ? What do you think ? Do you recognize yourself in Me and in My fears about you or Me ? And not to mention the unmentionable. You have "mucked around" with a child, with internet pedophilia and so on .... That child, it's actually you. You just forgot that. I'm your answer to the need to change, to dare do something else, to transform an important part of who you are. To realign you and Me or rather between you and you.

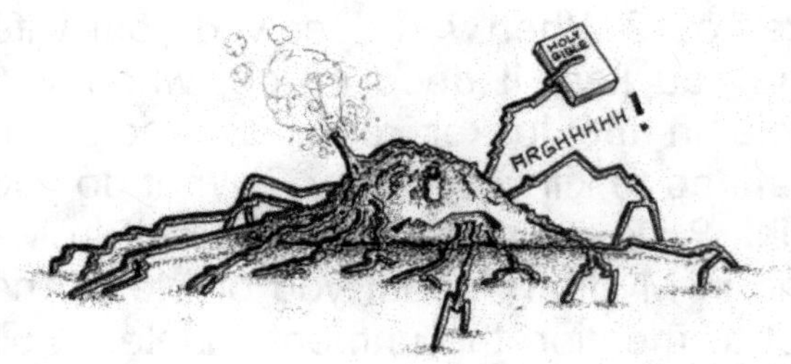

HOLY BIBLE
ARGHHHHH!

9 Death

Death, the grim reaper, the ghost, the eternal resting place ! We all go there! The one and only way out of life: had you forgotten that ? Relegated to other spaces and other times maybe be ? Have you thought about it ? What is death ? The big void, the leap of faith, the great departure, paradise or hell, limbo or Bardot, compost or dust or the crossing with the ferryman Anubis or even St Peter and the last judgment ... death fascinates and frightens.

When was the first time you met it ? And what effect did it have on you ? Or did you push "the thing", (note, we do not say the word death in our society), further away or did you lock it up like a skeleton or an unhealthy and ill-loved corpse in a cupboard ? Remember the death of that bird, that pigeon, when you were 7, you certainly do remember ? What did you do about all that ? What did the adults tell you ? What were your inner thoughts? When your grandfather or grandmother, that beloved dog departed, are they like wounds, deep in your heart or are you soothed about it all ? Do they visit you, from time in time, in your dreams or in a quiet moment in your everyday life ? Is there a life after life ? A big black hole ? A nothingness ? Especially a nothingness in your thought and this nothingness is connected to fear. Visit this nothingness ! you might be surprised ! Go and read my friend Raymond Moody, what I call a real doctor, he has understood many things and in addition he is such a nice man. Look at the phenomena of mediumship and communication with the afterlife. It's fascinating, and what's more, it opens the mind. From time immemorial it has existed. Today even more so as the veils between dimensions are thinning and lifting !

The film by Dieter Broers, an evolutionary physicist and scientist, bears witness to this. Take a look at the film "Mediums, from one world to another" in which you can see Clare. This woman has moved a great deal throughout her life. Take a little time to "visit" and explore, life, death. Feel the whole adventure and explore...You could also do it with a Dolores Cannon therapist, or other types of deep hypnotic states. You don't have to eat psychedelics to do so, although that may help.
Go ahead, dare ! I can assure you that it will help you.

Find a therapist and explore. The sooner you have integrated the notion of death, the sooner you will be able to live your life fully.

Know that there are some good American studies, on the use of psilocybin, a psycho active substance from a magical mushroom used traditionally by shamans around the world. This is to help you open other spaces and visions, when everything seems blocked to you. A very good book by the scientific journalist Michael Pollan talks about these studies. It could be very useful to unlock yourself and open your mind, gain a broader vision. These studies are rather promising. Remember shamans all over the world have known about all this for centuries.

Anyway, the bulk of your vision is so very narrow, so go ahead and open it up, you will be the winner!

What are you afraid of ?

9.1 Suffering, fatigue, pain and palliative care

What is suffering ? Take the definition of the Harrap's dictionary: "Suffering is a state of prolonged pain, distress or hardship."
It can also mean that one is particularly affected by various difficulties, sorrows, or unhappiness.
What is pain ? A painful, unpleasant sensation felt in a part of the body, caused by illness or injury.

My answer is simply for both: it is very complicated! You will have to dissociate your physical suffering and other pains from your psychological suffering (often totally self-inflicted) which is really made of another matter, especially that based on your moral code and your values. The moral code or your values are by definition questionable. They depend on your thought processes and your mind and of course your beliefs, your upbringing or the societal or religious background in which you grew up and where these codes came from. Take an example: you forget to celebrate your mother's birthday or Mother's Day: you leave in a state of anger or sadness (disease or distress) and you think that people do not love you and that it is always like that. You feel really down, angry or sad. Such celebrations are important values in our Western society. Did you know that the date of Mother's Day varies from one country to another ? that in many places it doesn't even exist. For France it was Napoleon's idea. Just a man and an idea !

So, free yourself from all this and you will no longer suffer from these elements. Or you stick to your old way of thinking and the suffering may be abominable. In the end it's up to you to choose and decide. What is important finally ? do you want to suffer ? The Buddhists would tell you that you created everything yourself because you are your thoughts. Have you thought about that ?

Emotional suffering is similar to psychic suffering, adding the possible phases of mourning, and emotional damage related to the phenomena of attachment and loss. For the phases of mourning, Dr. Kübler Ross summarizes them very well.

With regards to the pain and the suffering part of your physical body, it is related to life, not to your belief system but to your neuro-sensory system and your brain. A lesion is at the origin of a nervous message captured by the nerve endings, sorts of sentinels to this pain. This message is then transmitted by the nerve fibres to the brain, via the spinal cord: the relays of all nervous messages. So, it's something different to suffering. Of course, if you have too much physical pain you will enter a state of chronic suffering related to this.

Whatever happens, you will have to take care of your physical pain and your emotional and moral suffering. The physical pain can also be treated with your belief system and the help of your thoughts. Acupuncture, sophrology, creative visualization and conscious mind full meditation or other more oriental approaches, drugs, anaesthetics and psychotropic drugs, including opioids but also cannabis and methadone and entheogens (psychadelics) are possible approaches.

Surgical approaches and cerebral stimulators can also be considered, knowing that, there again, they are not an infallible approach and can bring their cohort of problems. Western medication such as anti-inflammatories (including cortisone) and synthetic analgesics are not to be dismissed of course, but should be used with great discernment.

There is no glory in suffering despite what your religions may have taught you, and that it would be a way of getting rid of some sort of sin ... NO !. The belief in expiation, still remains a powerful and punitive thought force. Look for all possible ways of treating yourself including those that work with your mind and your creative power of thought. You will not be able to move on far without having settled this strong biological part of you.

But do remember, that your body is talking to you. It also has things to tell you. From time to time, by highlighting one or another thing of your past, you will free yourself from the pain stored in your rather more cellular memory. A hypnosis session can also help you release more distant memories.

It would seem that I'm tiring you ? What is fatigue? ... Strange phenomenon ! Go and read a bit about it! You always imagine that you lack something, for example iron, that you are anemic, or that you lack this or that ... Have you ever imagined that the doctors' treatments may not be suitable for you, or are even toxic ? That your alignment within yourself is not ok ? That your surroundings are not good for you ? That

even the place where you live is toxic, overloaded, noisy, or unhealthy ? There are many other causes of your states of being that are not Me !
I love to laugh when you get upset and that's rather often. I would gladly give you a little prod...Then of course, I would laugh loudly ... Naughty ? Me ? No ! just a guardian.

Could you just be tired maybe ? Running around like a crazy headless chicken all day, all the time, everywhere and nowhere. Watching too much television and far too late, forgetting to breathe.
Did you realize that your breathing is faulty, or that you completely forgot to breathe ?
Many things tell you to calm down, to stop, to take time, to slow down. Where are you running to like this ? Furthermore you're running inside your head, you will quickly do this or that and looking into your overloaded diary. Whatever, I'm going to force you to slow down, and your body will do this too. It's Me, let's say, who is in command when you don't listen !

Preparing for your own death is very important. Read the subject up, observe your reactions and your emotions. When you have the opportunity to rub shoulders with it, do not run away. And do it as early as you can, the more you wait the less you will have choice, as it is an important part of life.

Know that the days before your death, when I have taken up all the room inside you, can be gentle, serene and calm. Ask to be accompanied by either those you love or by professionals, and even better both. Gentleness and love as well as therapeutic competence are good for you.

10 Conclusion

What I have to tell you whatever you do with me:

Start by deciding to change.

Take your life into your own hands.

Become the main actor of your life.

Learn to listen to yourself.

Identify the heart of the problem, therefore learn to clarify.

Become aware of the impact of what's bothering you in all areas of your life.

Clarify the cause of your difficulties.

Define precisely the goal (goals) you want to achieve in the given situation and in your life, and put your heart and soul into this.

Your intention must be absolutely clear.

Identify obstacles that prevent you from achieving your goal (goals).

Determine the concrete actions and steps that will help you gradually achieve, step by step, your goal (goals).

Let go of the final result, by taking small steps, one day at a time. All paths require patience and, above all, perseverance.

Surrender to other higher and benevolent forces if you feel the need to or when you no longer know what to think. These forces will help you no matter what your belief system is.

Me Cancer, I am first of all a thought-form. Even if I have an unfortunate tendency to be rather negative. The more you feed Me in my dark part, the more you give your power to that part - that of destroying you in the here and now and that is exactly what I do. It is in this, that I help you change and destroy the little you. If you give me that power, that's what I'll do, so take back your power. Imperatively, take back your power, one step at a time. No one can ever destroy the big You.

11 Suggested readings

Abraham Hicks channeled by Ester Hicks https://www.abraham-hicks.com/

Albert Einstein, physicist and philosopher, Energy is matter.

Alex Orbito *:* www.pyramidofasia.org
See also « les guérisseurs de la foi », Jean Dominique Michel – film, documentary in French
https://www.filmsdocumentaires.com/films/169-guerisseurs-philippins

Alexandro Jodorowsky : Guérir, c'est être soi | Psychologies.com voir article dans
www.psychologies.com

Anne Ancelin Schutzenberger (Pr) Aïe mes aïeux ISBN 2220040577 ; Ces enfants malades de leurs parents. Vouloir guérir : L'aide au malade atteint d'un cancer ISBN-13: 978-2228914413 Psychogénéalogie, trans-générationnelle

Anne-Marie Giraud (Dr) Huiles essentiels et cancer www.drgiraudannemarie.fr

Alice Miller the body never lies ISBN-13: 978-0393328639

Allison Drummond, cured from stage 4 cancer without chemo or radiation, conference in English https://instantteleseminar.com/Events/108320025

Association Suisse pour le suicide assisté : Swiss association for assisted suicide
1) Association EXIT www.exit-geneve.ch
2) Association Dignitas
   www.dignitas.ch

En France, mouvement important mais PAS de suicide assisté, ni d'euthanasie. Chacun aura à faire son petit bout pour permettre un jour, peut-être, sûrement. https://www.admd.net

La Belgique est ouverte à l'euthanasie depuis 2002 https://www.francebleu.fr/.../euthanasie-en-belgique-le-recours-pour-les-patients-francais-1507284876

Bashar channeled by Darryl Anka https://www.bashar.org

Bernie Siegel (Dr) Love, medicine and miracles ISBN-13: 978-0060919832
 berniesiegelmd.com/

Bert Hellinger: Family Constellations: A Practical Guide to Uncovering the Origins of Family Conflict ISBN-13: 978-1556438325
www.bert-hellinger.com

Breuss cure of
https://cancer.ooreka.fr › Prévention et traitements
www.guerir.org
Rudolf Breuss cancer cure correctly applied: Guide to cancer treatment ISBN-13: 978-1511969741

Bruce Lipton : Biology of belief ISBN-13: 978-1401952471
Epigenetics and the power of your mind
https://www.youtube.com/watch?v=PCYPKsI4xNQ
https://www.youtube.com/watch?v=abwHFLcLWZ4
https://www.brucelipton.com/

Candace Pert (Dr)
https://www.inrees.com
Molecules of Emotion: Why You Feel The Way You Feel, ISBN-13: 978-0671033972

Cannabis as pain treatment; cannabis oil
https://realfarmacy.com/spanish-study-confirms-cannabis-oil-cures

https://www.principesactifs.org/spain-
study-confirms-cannabis-oil-
https://www.ncbi.nlm.nih.gov/pmc/article
s/PMC4791148/

System of help for patients in USA
https://thesacredplant.com

CBD oil in Switzerland:
https://swissmedicalcannabis.ch
www.alchimiaweb.com

Carl Gustave Jung (Dr).
Man in search of the soul ISBN-13: 978-
1684220908
https://www.jung.de

Carl Simonton (Dr) The healing journey;
Centre Simonton, in Switzerland,
Lausanne www.simonton.ch/fr

Catherine Kousmine (Dr): Sauvez votre
corps, Éditions Robert Laffont, 1987,
(ISBN 2290336327). Only in French.
Fondation Kousmine, Switzerland :
www.solvida.org

Christian Boukaram (Pr) Le pouvoir anti
cancer des émotions
ASIN: B01B98PSJ4
In French or in Spanish
drboukaram.com/dr-boukaram

Christian Tal Schaller (Dr) .... Youtube «le tigre »
https://www.youtube.com/watch?v=OgJLUjB2t-M
Only in french

Clare Munday (Dr) et Sylvie Blanchon
Cancer et sens de la vie
https://www.amazon.fr/Dr-Clare-Munday/e/B078JHW27G only in French
www.drclaremunday.ch

David Servan Schreiber (Dr)
www.guerir.org
Anti-cancer ISBN-13: 978-2266215794
Anticancer ISBN-13: 978-2221108710

Denise Gilliand Médiums le livre ISBN-13: 978-2828912475, film/DVD
www.mediums-lefilm.com

Dieter Broers, German physicist, changes induced by the sun. Solar Revolution: Why Mankind Is on the cusp of an Evolutionary Leap ISBN-13: 978-1583945049
www.solar-revolution-movie.com
https://dieter-broers.de

Dione Fortune Psychic Self-Defense, ISBN-13: 978-1578635092

Dolores Cannon QHHT,

quantum therapy deep hypnosis
https://www.qhhtofficial.com/
https://dolorescannon.com/

Dominique Belpomme (Pr) : French
oncologist in Paris, effects of
electromagnetic waves on health.
Only French
https://www.santemagazine.fr
Actualités
https://www.youtube.com/watch?v=dgAF
vHaBa1c

Gregg Braden
https://www.greggbraden.com

Gerson cure
https://gerson.org/gerpress/the-gerson-
therapy/

Helen Schucman and William Thetford
A course in miracles ISBN-13: 978-
0976420057

Henri Joyeux (Pr) :
https://professeur-joyeux.com
Changez d'alimentation ISBN-13: 978-
2266261777- Only in French

Hulda Clark :
A cure for all diseases ISBN-13: 978-
1890035013

The cure for all cancers ISBN-13: 978-
0963632821
drclark-france.com;
https://www.drclark.net/en-us/

Iscador, treatment with mistletoe
https://www.iscador.com/

Jean Seignalet (Dr) Only in French
Alimentation ou la troisième médecine
ISBN-13: 978-2268074009
https://www.seignalet.fr/fr

John of god Brazilian healer
https://en.wikipedia.org/wiki/Jo%C3%A3
o_de_Deus_(medium)
www.joaodedeus-jeandedieu.com

Les miracles de Lourdes : la science
face à la foi, Philippe Aziz Robert
Lafont ASIN: B00C2TFJDU Only in
French

Lise Bourbeau :
Heal your wounds and find your true self
ISBN: 978-2920932210
https://www.lisebourbeau.com

Interesting books /Only in French

La princesse qui croyait aux contes de fées Marcia Graad

Le Tueur de dragons au coeur lourd Marcia Grad Powers, François Minaudier: ISBN: 9782940500055

Le chevalier à l'armure rouillée Robert Fisher, Ambre Eds

Luc Montagnier (Pr) prix Nobel de médecine 2008, Virus du sida - Only in French
https://www.youtube.com/watch?v=dgAFvHaBa1c
https://www.inrees.com/articles/memoire-eau-revolution/
https://www.youtube.com/watch?v=yo6B7ggkOo0

Masaru Emoto: The hidden Messages in Water ISBN-13: 978-1416522195

Methadone in cancer, University of Ulm, Dr Claudia Friesen- German
Email: methadone-krebs@uni-ulm.de

https://www.ligue-cancer.net/forum/38792_chimiotherapie-plus-efficace-avec-racemate-de-d-l-methadone   only in French

Michael Greger (Dr)
https://nutritionfacts.org

Michael Pollan
https://michaelpollan.com
https://www.youtube.com/watch?v=Whm
nx_Cb5ts
How to change your mind. ISBN
9781594204227
www.maps.org/research

Peter Arthur Straubinger : Lumière
Austrian documentary film 2010.
https://lightdocumentary.space/tag/peter-
arthur-straubinger/

Placebo / nocebo effects
https://www.ncbi.nlm.nih.gov/pubmed/24
909245

Kübler Ross Elisabeth (Dr) ; The stages
of grief, On death and dying ISBN-13:
978-0020891307;
La mort est un nouveau soleil : Quand la
mort est une porte ouverte sur une autre
vie ISBN-13: 978-2266122191

Raymond Moody
https://www.inrees.com/articles/La-vie-
apres-la-vie-les-premieres-analyses-de-
Raymond-Moody/
Life after life
www.lifeafterlife.com

Rupert Sheldrake: a new life science; morphogenetiques fields or morphic fields ; https://www.sheldrake.org/

Steiner Rudolf (Dr), philosopher writer, Antroposophy – Iscador
Lukas Klinik, Arlesheim, Switzerland: clinic specialised in cancer ; https://www.klinik-arlesheim.ch

Thierry Lestrade Le jeûne, une nouvelle thérapie ? livre Poche, ISBN-13: 978-2707188175- only in French

Vitamine C : Linus Pauling
https://www.cancer.gov/about-cancer/treatment/cam/patient/vitamin-c-pdq
www.traitement-du-cancer.fr/ in French

www.ingramcontent.com/pod-product-compliance
Lightning Source LLC
Chambersburg PA
CBHW061710250726
48657CB00002B/584